POCKET SERIES FOR MRCP PART II

BOOK 2

Gastroenterology, Endocrinology and Renal Medicine

POCKET SERIES FOR MRCP PART II

BOOK 2
Gastroenterology, Endocrinology and Renal Medicine

Edited by Richard L. Hawkins MBBS FRCS

Gastroenterology:
David Maxton MD MRCP
University Hospital of South Manchester

Endocrinology:
Ah Wah Chan MBCh MRCP
Gareth Williams MA MD MRCP
Royal Liverpool Hospital

Renal Medicine:
Ian Barton MA MRCP
St Thomas' Hospital, London

PASTEST

© 1990 PASTEST SERVICE
Cranford Lodge, Bexton Road, Knutsford
Cheshire WA16 0ED
Tel: 0565 55226

First printed in 1990

British Library Cataloguing in Publication Data

MRCP Part 2 Pocket Books
   1. Gastroenterology, endocrinology and renal medicine
   I. Hawkins, Richard 1949–   II. Series
   610

ISBN 0–906896–42–8

Text prepared by Turner Associates, Knutsford, Cheshire.
Phototypeset by Speedset Ltd, Ellesmere Port, Cheshire.
Printed in Great Britain by Billing and Sons, Worcester.

CONTENTS

Answers and teaching notes are on
the reverse of each question page.

BIBLIOGRAPHY

GASTROENTEROLOGY
  Diseases of the Liver and Biliary System. S. Sherlock. 7th ed.
    1985 Blackwell Scientific.
  Oxford Textbook of Medicine. Weatherall et al. 2nd ed.
    1987 Oxford University Press.
  Textbook of Medicine. R. L. Souhami and J. Moxham. (Gastro-
    enterology section by Beck and Long) 1990 Churchill Livingstone.

ENDOCRINOLOGY
  Basic and Clinical Endocrinology. Edited by F. Greenspan
    and P. Forsham. 2nd ed. 1986 Lange Medical Publications.
  Endocrinology: A logical approach for clinicians. W. Jubiz
    2nd ed. 1987 McGraw Hill.

RENAL MEDICINE
  Nephrology Pocket Consultant. P. E. Gower. 2nd ed.
    1990 Blackwell Scientific.

INTRODUCTION

The MRCP Part 2 Examination is a test of competent clinical practice as opposed to the theoretical knowledge required for Part 1. The examiners want to be reassured that the candidate is professional in his or her approach and manner, accomplished in technique, safe in practice and honest in ignorance. There is no doubt that efficient, systematic preparation for the Part 2 can make all the difference between passing and failing the examination. Familiarity with the type of questions being set, together with a knowledge of how best to present the answers and how they are marked by the examiners, will all help candidates to do their best in the examination.

Each of these three PasTest pocket books contain sample case histories and data interpretations carefully written and edited by doctors involved in the teaching and preparation of candidates for the MRCP examination. The case material, data and questions presented have all been chosen for their similarity to those experienced in recent official examinations:

    Book 1: Cardiology and Respiratory Medicine
    Book 2: Gastroenterology, Endocrinology and Renal Medicine
    Book 3: Haematology, Rheumatology and Neurology.

The best way to use these books is to work through each question in a methodical manner keeping to the time limits set by the Royal College. This will give useful practice in coming to quick decisions about the answers, which can then be looked up, corrected and thought about in a more leisurely manner.

By working through these books and studying the correct answers and teaching notes, a candidate will be able to pinpoint specific topics and subject areas where further reading and study would be beneficial before the examination. **Please note that the correct answers given in these books are not presented in a simple list as required by the College on examination day, but are incorporated within the teaching notes.**

The written section of the examination consists of three question papers:

(a) Case Histories (four or more compulsory questions in 55 minutes.)
(b) Data Interpretation (ten compulsory questions in 45 minutes.)
(c) Projected Material (twenty compulsory questions in 40 minutes.)

The Royal College has published a booklet of 2 past MRCP Part 2 written examinations (general medicine and paediatrics) and all candidates would be wise to be familiar with these, in particular the simple answer format preferred.

Introduction

Advice on How to Answer the Questions

The written part of the MRCP Part 2 examination has been designed to require minimal writing so that maximum time may be devoted by the candidate to thinking through the problems presented while, at the same time, it allows for objective marking by the examiners. This means that marks are awarded by the examiners in a predetermined manner. Specific answers are required and so candidates must listen carefully to the invigilator's instructions and understand exactly how to present their answers. Since specific answers are required, it is of no use to treat the questions as short answer questions in which you attempt to explain your thoughts to the examiner. Answers should be precise, yet complete, in their meaning. Vague answers score significantly lower marks.

Each question asks for a specific number of answers. Correct answers to a question will receive maximum marks but since there may be more than one possible correct answer, marks will be awarded on a scale according to their acceptibility. Where the 'best' answer is much better than the others, the difference in marking between the best and the other answers will be greater. Answers in excess of the number requested will be ignored. For example, if three diagnoses are given instead of two, only the first two will be marked, even if the third represents the best response. Space is given in the examination paper for each of your answers and it will be of considerable help to the examiners if you confine your answers to one per line.

All three papers in the written section are ascribed the same maximum number of marks. The final score for each candidate is the aggregate mark of all three papers. In order to pass, it is not necessary therefore to obtain a pass mark in each of the three papers, so long as the aggregate mark reaches the required pass mark.

Candidates who pass the written section are invited to attend for further examination in the clinical and oral sections. Those who marginally fail the written section may also proceed to the clinical and oral sections but, to succeed in the examination as a whole, have to obtain additional marks in these last two sections.

Candidates who have clearly failed the written section are deemed to have failed the examination as a whole and must resit the written section in order to proceed in the examination.

It is hoped that the material provided in these three pocket books will prove instrumental in the success of many Part 2 candidates.

viii

1. A 32 year old homosexual man is known to be HIV positive. He complains of severe retrosternal discomfort and dysphagia. Symptomatic treatment helps this symptom to some extent but 6 months later he returns with severe watery diarrhoea without blood, associated with griping abdominal pain. Prolonged recovery occurs but he remains underweight. One year later he returns with papilloedema and a dense right hemiplegia.

Questions:

1. Give three possible causes of the initial retrosternal pain.

2. Give four likely causes for diarrhoea in this patient.

3. What is the most likely cause for the hemiplegia?

Answers overleaf

1. 1. Oral and oesophageal involvement in AIDS patients is common. Herpes simplex, candidiasis or cytomegalovirus infection are likely pathogens in the oesophagus. Aphthous ulceration can also involve the oesophagus.

2. Diarrhoea is frequent in AIDS with many possible pathogens. Cryptosporidium, giardiasis and cytomegalovirus are likely but salmonella and shigella species together with campylobacter may also complicate the condition. Atypical mycobacteria and the AIDS virus itself may also cause intestinal damage.

3. The most probable cause of an intra-cerebral space occupying lesion in this man is toxoplasmosis.

2. A 20 year old man presents with longstanding diarrhoea and abdominal pain of more recent onset. The abdominal pain is colicky in nature and mostly in the right iliac fossa. He has been diagnosed as suffering from cystic fibrosis but attends outpatients infrequently. While in hospital for investigation he has a haematemesis and melaena requiring a four unit blood transfusion.

Questions:

1. What is the most likely cause for the diarrhoea?

2. Give two possible causes for the abdominal pain.

3. Suggest the most likely reason for the gastrointestinal haemorrhage.

Answers overleaf

2. 1. <u>Pancreatic insufficiency with steatorrhoea</u> is a common manifestation of <u>cystic fibrosis</u> in the gut and is likely to explain the diarrhoea.

2. Poorly controlled steatorrhoea may lead to a mass of partially digested food producing sub-acute small bowel obstruction. This is known as '<u>meconium ileus equivalent</u>'. <u>The incidence of gallstones is also increased in cystic fibrosis.</u>

3. <u>Liver cirrhosis complicates older sufferers. Haemorrhage is probably from oesophageal varices.</u>

3. A 67 year old woman has a long history of Crohn's disease. She is admitted with severe weight loss and general debility. Abdominal pain and torrential diarrhoea have been present for several months. She has had multiple bowel resections in the past. Current therapy consists only of vitamin B_{12} and folic acid supplements. Examination shows a thin and cachetic woman with marked muscle wasting. The muscles particularly of the thighs are so weak she has difficulty walking. Multiple scars are present on abdominal examination.

Questions:

1. Give five possible causes for the diarrhoea in this case.

2. Suggest two useful investigations to elucidate the most probable diagnosis.

3. Suggest a possible reason for the muscle weakness found in this patient.

Answers overleaf

3. 1. <u>Short bowel syndrome</u> is a potential explanation of the diarrhoea. Alternative diagnoses are <u>recurrent Crohn's disease</u> or possibly a <u>complicating entero-enteric fistula. An abscess is less likely. A specific intestinal infection is possible or bacterial overgrowth in the small intestine. Bile salt malabsorption after terminal ileal resection is another possibility.</u>

    2. A <u>small bowel enema or follow through</u> may delineate active Crohn's disease or show an intestinal fistula. A <u>colonoscopy</u> may also confirm active inflammatory bowel disease. <u>Ultrasound is less useful but could confirm an abscess.</u>

    3. The predominantly <u>proximal myopathy</u> suggests the possibility <u>of osteomalacia</u>.

4. A 48 year old Chinese man is known to be HBsAg positive. He is being followed up yearly in the clinic when his liver function tests begin to deteriorate. The bilirubin level is elevated and jaundice deepens. Ascites develops together with abdominal pain. He is then admitted as an emergency having become confused at home over the previous week. A diagnosis of hepatic encephalopathy is made. Two days after admission however you are called to see him because he has deteriorated suddenly. On arrival he is unrousable but pulse and blood pressure are normal. Rectal examination is also normal and there is no evidence of haematemesis.

Questions:

1. Give four possible causes for the deterioration in liver function tests.

2. Suggest four possible causes for the development of hepatic encephalopathy.

3. Give two likely reasons for the sudden final reduction in conscious level.

Answers overleaf

4. 1. Deterioration of liver disease in an HBsAg carrier suggests complication by delta virus superinfection or development of hepatoma. Hepatic damage from drugs, alcohol or another type of hepatitis should be considered. Simple progression of the liver damage may also explain the deterioration.

2. Hepatic encephalopathy may be precipitated by infection particularly ascitic infection. Drugs may also precipitate coma as may rapid fluid loss due to diuretic therapy. Electrolyte disturbance, gastrointestinal haemorrhage and constipation are other possible causes.

3. Sudden deterioration in conscious level suggests inappropriate sedation frequently with opiates or hypoglycaemia. Cerebral oedema is a frequent terminal event in such patients and should be considered.

5. A 14 year old boy is admitted with a haematemesis. Previously he has generally been well. There is no past history of abdominal pain, drug ingestion or jaundice except after birth when he suffered from severe haemolytic disease of the newborn. On examination he is not jaundiced but has an enlarged spleen. Acute upper gastrointestinal endoscopy showed prominent oesophageal varices. A liver biopsy is reported as normal. Regular injection sclerotherapy is commenced and after eight treatments his oesophageal varices are insignificant. However he is again admitted with a large haematemesis.

Questions:

1. What is the most probable cause for his oesophageal varices?

2. Suggest the most likely site of bleeding for his second haematemesis.

Answers overleaf

5. 1. The history suggests a <u>portal vein thrombosis</u> probably second-ary to umbilical vein catheterisation in the neonatal period.

  2. Once <u>oesophageal varices have been eradicated bleeding may still occur from gastric varices</u>.

6. A 28 year old man suffers from severe haemophilia A. He is admitted to hospital on this occasion with abdominal and back pain which came on after a minor fall at work. The pain is located particularly in the right loin but there is no haematuria. On examination he is distressed and in pain. Abdominal examination reveals no guarding or tenderness but back movements are limited.

While in hospital it is noted that his liver function tests are mildly abnormal. Upper gastrointestinal endoscopy shows oesophageal varices and a liver biopsy establishes cirrhosis.

Questions:

1. What is the most likely cause of his original presentation?

2. Suggest the most probable aetiology for the liver disease.

Answers overleaf

6. 1. The likelihood is that this man has had another bleed. The history is suggestive of a retroperitoneal site, possibly the psoas muscle.

   2. Cirrhosis is common in haemophiliacs who have received Factor VIII treatment. The most probable aetiology is non-A non-B hepatitis although hepatitis B is also possible.

7. A 27 year old woman is seen in out-patients. She complains of colicky abdominal pains partly relieved by defaecation. She has diarrhoea, passing up to five motions per day associated with mucus, but no blood. She also described the sensation of rectal dissatisfaction. Her other main symptom is of visible abdominal distension and bloating particularly towards the end of the day. Otherwise her general health is good and she has not lost any weight.

After attending the clinic for several months she is re-referred by her GP with changed symptoms of epigastric pain after meals with nausea and a feeling of early satiety.

Questions:

1. What is the most probable diagnosis?

2. List four factors in the history which support your diagnosis.

3. What is the most likely cause of her upper gastrointestinal symptoms?

Answers overleaf

7. 1. By far the most common disease to produce these symptoms in a young woman is <u>irritable bowel syndrome</u>.

    2. The positive factors in the history suggesting the above diagnosis are the <u>abdominal bloating</u>, the <u>relief of pain on defaecation</u>, the <u>presence of mucus in the stools</u> and <u>rectal dissatisfaction</u>. Negative features are the <u>lack of weight loss</u> or <u>blood in the stools.</u>

    3. <u>Upper gastrointestinal symptoms are frequent in irritable bowel syndrome and are usually categorised as non-ulcer dyspepsia.</u>

1. A 54 year old man complains of episodic diarrhoea. He has a history of recurrent pulmonary infections and sinusitis over the last three years. There are no abnormal findings on examination.

Results include:

Hb	13.4 g/dl
WBC	6.0 x 10^9/l
Platelets	267 x 10^9/l

Serum	bilirubin	17	μmol/l
	alkaline phosphatase	110 iu/l	
	aspartate transaminase	30 iu/l	
	albumin	42 g/l	
	total protein	61 g/l	
	globulin	19 g/l	
	IgG	4 g/l (normal 8–16)	
	IgA	0.2 g/l (normal 1.2–4.0)	
	IgM	0.2 g/l (normal 0.5–1.6)	

HIV test: negative

Questions:

1. What is the most likely diagnosis?
2. Give one alternative diagnosis.
3. Give two possible reasons for the diarrhoea.

2. A fit 24 year old soldier has the following liver blood tests on routine testing:

Serum	bilirubin	38 μmol/l
	alkaline phosphatase	90 iu/l
	aspartate transaminase	32 iu/l

No bilirubin is detectable in the urine.

Questions:

1. Suggest the most likely reason for these results.
2. Give one differential diagnosis.
3. Suggest two methods of confirming your diagnosis.

Answers overleaf

1. 1. All the immunoglobulins are reduced. In a patient of this age the most likely diagnosis is common variable or acquired hypo-gammaglobulinaemia.

2. Lymphoma should be considered as an alternative.

3. Intestinal infection is the common reason for diarrhoea in these cases, particularly giardiasis and bacterial overgrowth. An inflammatory colitis may also occur.

2. 1. The results suggest Gilbert's syndrome with the features of an unconjugated hyperbilirubinaemia with normal liver blood tests.

2. The major alternative diagnosis is of chronic haemolysis.

3. The diagnosis may be confirmed by demonstrating a rise in serum bilirubin on fasting or after intravenous nicotinic acid.

3. A 36 year old man is admitted to hospital with jaundice, fever and abdominal pain. Tender hepatomegaly was present on examination. However there was no history of haematemesis or melaena or signs of bleeding on examination.

   The following blood tests were obtained:

Hb	4.8 g/dl
MCV	140 fl
WBC	9.8×10^9/l
Platelets	155×10^9/l

Serum		
	bilirubin	242 µmol/l
	alkaline phosphatase	157 iu/l
	aspartate aminotransferase	480 iu/l
	gamma-glutamyl transpeptidase	410 iu/l

   Questions:

   1. What is the most likely cause of this patient's liver disease?

   2. Suggest three possible causes for the anaemia.

4. A 64 year old man suffered a cardiac arrest but was successfully resuscitated. Four days later the following results were obtained:

Serum		
	bilirubin	70 µmol/l
	alkaline phosphatase	245 iu/l
	aspartate transaminase	2500 iu/l

   Question:

   1. What is the likely diagnosis?

Answers overleaf
17

3. 1. Acute alcoholic hepatitis is the most likely reason for the liver disease particularly with this degree of macrocytosis.

   2. Anaemia with macrocytosis in alcoholic liver disease may be due to a direct effect of alcohol on haemopoiesis. In this case acute folate deficiency and haemolysis should also be considered. Vitamin B_{12} deficiency is also a possibility.

4. 1. The history and the vast rise in aspartate aminotransferase levels are suggestive of ischaemic hepatitis due to anoxic damage occurring at the time of the cardiac arrest.

5. A 24 year old woman presents to an infertility clinic complaining of amenorrhoea. She has been well apart from recurrent urinary tract infections. She is obese and has spider naevi.
Investigations show:

Hb   11.7 g/dl
WBC   4.3 x 10^9/l
Platelets 120 x 10^9/l

Serum calcium   2.20 mmol/l
           phosphate   1.1 mmol/l
           total protein   86 g/l
           albumin   32 g/l
           bilirubin   90 μmol/l
           alkaline phosphatase   193 iu/l
           aspartate aminotransaminase   500 iu/l

Questions:

1. What is the most likely diagnosis?
2. List four factors which support your diagnosis.
3. List four other possible diagnoses.
4. Give four important investigations to help in the differential diagnosis.

6. A 54 year old man gives a four-month history of diarrhoea with weight loss of five kilograms.
Investigations show:

Hb   14.3 g/dl
WBC   8.0 x 10^9/l
Serum bilirubin   20 μmol/l
           albumin   36 g/l
           alkaline phosphatase   134 iu/l
           aspartate transaminase   60 iu/l

3-day faecal fat excretion: 60 mmol/day
25 g oral D-xylose: 24% recovery after 5 hours.

Questions:

1. What is the most likely diagnosis?
2. List three possible underlying causes of this condition.
3. Suggest two useful investigations.

Answers overleaf

5. 1. <u>Autoimmune chronic active hepatitis</u> is the most likely diagnosis.

  2. <u>Female sex</u> and her <u>age</u> make the above diagnosis very likely. <u>Spider naevi</u> and <u>amenorrhoea are also characteristic features</u>. <u>The serum globulins</u> (obtained by subtracting the albumin from the total protein) <u>are increased</u>, also a feature of chronic active hepatitis.

  3. <u>Viral hepatitis</u>, either <u>acute or chronic, is a possibility</u>. <u>Drug-induced liver disease should be considered perhaps in this case due to nitrofurantoin</u>. <u>Wilson's disease, alcoholic liver damage, primary biliary cirrhosis and alpha-1-antitrypsin deficiency are included in the differential diagnosis</u>. <u>Extrahepatic biliary obstruction should always be excluded</u>.

  4. Many investigations are possible but <u>HBsAG</u> and an <u>auto-immune screen, in particular the anti-nuclear and anti-smooth muscle antibodies are essential</u>. <u>Liver biopsy should also be performed and bile duct obstruction excluded by ultrasound</u>.

6. 1. The <u>faecal fat excretion is high but the D-xylose excretion is normal</u>. This combination suggests <u>chronic pancreatitis</u>.

  2. The most likely cause in a man of this age is <u>alcohol abuse</u>. Other possibilities include <u>biliary disease particularly gallstones, or acute pancreatitis especially if complicated by abscess or pseudocyst</u>. <u>Hypercalcaemia, hyperlipaemia, trauma, malnutrition</u> and <u>haemochromatosis</u> are rarer causes. There is also an association with <u>primary biliary cirrhosis</u> and <u>sclerosing cholangitis</u>. <u>Pancreatic cancer requires exclusion</u>.

  3. A plain <u>abdominal X-ray</u> is easy and may reveal pancreatic calcification. Further tests evaluate either pancreatic structure or function. Structural tests include <u>retrograde pancreatography (ERCP)</u> which is probably the most accurate and <u>CT scanning and ultrasound</u>. Oral function tests include <u>urinary para-aminobenzoic acid excretion and triolein breath tests while duodenal intubation is required for Lundh test meal or hormone stimulation tests</u>.

7. A 40 year old man presents with a two-week history of increasing painless jaundice. He has previously been well apart from occasional episodes of bloody diarrhoea which have never been investigated and low backache attributed to an industrial injury.

    The following results are obtained:

Serum	bilirubin	90 μmol/l
	alkaline phosphatase	850 iu/l
	aspartate transaminase	38 iu/l
	albumin	34 g/l

    Questions:

    1. What is the most likely diagnosis?
    2. How would you confirm this?
    3. Suggest three other investigations to help in the diagnosis?

8. A 46 year old woman is admitted with jaundice, gross ascites and peripheral oedema. The following results are obtained:

Plasma	sodium	120 mmol/l
	potassium	3.5 mmol/l
	urea	19.0 mmol/l
Serum	creatinine	320 μmol/l
	calcium	2.10 mmol/l
	phosphate	1.0 mmol/l
	total protein	59 g/l
	albumin	26 g/l
	bilirubin	479 μmol/l
	alkaline phosphatase	479 iu/l
	aspartate transaminase	147 iu/l
Blood glucose		6.0 mmol/l

Urinary sodium concentration:	7 mmol/l
Urinary osmolality:	305 mosm/l

    Questions:

    1. Give three possible causes for the impairment of renal function.
    2. Which do you consider the most likely underlying cause? Give two reasons for your decision.

Answers overleaf

7. 1. The history is suggestive of sclerosing cholangitis complicating ulcerative colitis.

    2. Endoscopic retrograde cholangio-pancreatography (ERCP) is the investigation of choice.

    3. Rectal or colonic biopsy might confirm ulcerative colitis and X-ray of the pelvis might also confirm the clinical suspicion of sacro-iliitis. The most useful liver investigation would be to exclude extra-hepatic biliary obstruction by ultrasound.

8. 1. Hepato-renal failure, acute tubular necrosis and dehydration are all possibilities in this situation complicating liver failure.

    2. Hepato-renal failure or 'functional' renal impairment is probably the commonest cause and the most likely in this case. This diagnosis is suggested by the low urinary sodium (below 12 mmol/l) whereas in acute tubular necrosis the urinary sodium is high. Dehydration would produce a concentrated urine with a urine/plasma osmolality ratio greater than 1.15. In this case the urine/plasma ratio is 1.12 (305/272 mosm/l).

9. A 34 year old man attending gastroenterology outpatients with Crohn's disease has the following results:

    Hb   13.9 g/dl
    PCV   0.42
    RBC $4.33 \times 10^{12}/l$
    WBC $2.1 \times 10^{9}/l$
    Platelets $98 \times 10^{9}/l$

Questions:

1. Suggest the most likely cause for these results?

10. A 63 year old man presents with a two-month history of dysphagia. Barium swallow suggests a smooth stricture at the gastro-oesophageal junction and the following report was obtained after oesophageal manometry:

The resting gastro-oesophageal sphincter pressure is increased and the sphincter fails to relax with swallowing. After swallowing there are no progressive peristaltic contractions with all contractions occurring simultaneously.

Questions:

1. What diagnosis does this report suggest?

2. What is the single most important alternative diagnosis in this case?

9. 1. Both the white blood count and the platelets are reduced. The most likely cause is treatment with azathioprine (Imuran). Haematological abnormalities also occur with sulphasalazine (Salazopyrin) including Heinz body anaemia, methaemoglobinaemia and haemolytic anaemia.

10. 1. The manometric features are suggestive of achalasia.

2. The rapid onset of symptoms in a man of this age together with the manometry findings are suspicious of pseudo-achalasia. This may be caused by malignancy at the gastro-oesophageal junction, often carcinoma of the cardia. Oesophageal amyloid, Riley-Day syndrome and Chagas disease are rare possibilities.

11. A 33 year old man underwent jejunal biopsy by Crosby capsule. The following results were obtained for intestinal disaccharidase activity:

	Specific activity (U/g protein)	(Normal range)
Maltase	27.46	130–456
Sucrase	33.84	40–152
Trehalase	3.19	10–80
Lactase	1.07	6–55

Questions:

1. What is the most likely diagnosis?

2. What is the most common abnormality of intestinal disaccharidase activity found in adults in the UK?

12. A 40 year old woman is found to have hepatomegaly on routine examination at a Well-Woman clinic.

The following results are obtained:

Hb 13.4 g/dl
WBC 6.4 x 10^9/l
ESR 4 mm in the first hour

Serum	bilirubin	5 μmol/l
	alkaline phosphatase	107 iu/l
	aspartate aminotransferase	22 iu/l

Ultrasound report: there is a single solid space occupying lesion in the left lobe of the liver. The remaining liver parenchyma looks normal.

Questions:

1. Suggest three possible causes for this appearance.

2. Suggest three non-invasive tests to attempt to distinguish between your possibilities.

Answers overleaf

11. 1. All four disaccharidases show reduced activity suggesting a generalised mucosal defect. Villous atrophy is the commonest cause usually secondary to coeliac disease.

2. Primary or racially determined lactase deficiency occurs in around 10% of Caucasian adults but in over 90% of non-Caucasians and is therefore the most common disaccharidase defect found in the UK.

12. 1. Focal single non-cystic liver masses are frequently solitary secondary tumours, primary liver tumours or haemangiomas. The normal liver blood tests might suggest a benign lesion.

2. Before more invasive procedures a plain chest X-ray may show primary or other secondary tumours. HBsAG and alpha feto-protein levels should be measured to diagnose primary liver tumour. A CT scan with contrast might also be helpful.

13. A 43 year old woman presented with diarrhoea.

The following results were obtained:

3-day faecal fat	30 mmol/day
jejunal biopsy	subtotal villous atrophy

A gluten free diet was started but after 12 months the diarrhoea persisted.

The following results were obtained:

3-day faecal fat	27 mmol/day
jejunal biopsy	subtotal villous atrophy

Questions:

1. What is the most likely explanation for the failure to respond to gluten withdrawal?
2. Give two alternative possible reasons.

14. An 86 year old lady is admitted with a two-month history of fever, weight loss and abdominal distension. There is no other relevant medical history. Examination reveals ascites.

The following results were obtained:

Hb   10.2 g/dl
WBC 15.0×10^9/l
ESR 70 mm in the first hour

Serum bilirubin   30 μmol/l
       alkaline phosphatase   147 iu/l
       aspartate aminotransferase   60 iu/l
Ascitic fluid: lymphocytes + +, no polymorphs,
               no organisms seen,
               protein 35 g/l

Questions

1. Suggest three possible diagnoses.
2. Suggest three other useful further investigations.

Answers overleaf
27

13. 1. By far the most common reason for a poor response to gluten withdrawal is failure to adhere to the diet, although this may be inadvertent.

2. Other rarer possibilities include an intestinal malignancy, for example lymphoma, complicating the coeliac disease, or the presence of an intestinal stricture or jejuno-ileitis. True resistant coeliac disease is rare. It is also possible the initial diagnosis was incorrect and another cause of subtotal villous atrophy has been overlooked.

14. 1. The high ascitic protein concentration and the presence of lymphocytes suggests tuberculous peritonitis or malignant disease. Cirrhosis of the liver is still possible but pancreatic ascites less likely.

2. Cytological investigation of the ascitic fluid for malignant cells is essential.

Culture of the fluid for bacterial and tuberculous infection should also be performed.

The possibility of tuberculous peritonitis may require peritoneoscopy to obtain histology. This procedure may also be diagnostic of malignant disease.

Further special investigations to consider would include liver ultrasound or CT and liver biopsy for malignant disease or cirrhosis. In ascites of pancreatic origin ascitic fluid amylase is usually raised.

1. A 32 year old previously healthy woman presented with a one-year history of palpitations, sweating, heat intolerance and intermittent diarrhoea. She had lost 5 kg in weight despite a good appetite. Her only medication was a low-dose oestrogen contraceptive pill. Her niece had neonatal hypothyroidism.

    Physical examination revealed an anxious woman with a pulse rate of 120/min, BP 120/80 mm Hg. She had a fine tremor of the hands with moist, warm palms. There was no lid lag or exophthalmos. The thyroid was diffusely enlarged without nodules and there was no cervical lymphadenopathy. All reflexes were generally brisk, but there were no other neurological abnormalities. Examination was otherwise unremarkable.

    Investigations showed:

FBC	normal
Plasma urea and electrolytes	normal
Blood glucose (random)	4.3 mmol/l
Serum albumin	43 g/l
Liver function tests	normal

    Thyroid function tests:

Total serum thyroxine	>220 nmol/l (normal range 60–160)
Free triiodothyronine (FT3)	13.1 pmol/l (normal range 2.9–8.9)
Free thyroxine (FT4)	32.3 pmol/l (normal range 9–24.5)
Serum thyrotrophin (TSH)	9.3 mU/l (normal range 0.5–5.5)

    Thyroid microsomal and thyroglobulin autoantibodies: absent
    Pertechnetate radio-isotope thyroid scan: diffuse enlargement and thyroid uptake of 18.9% at 20 minutes (normal range <3%)

Questions:

1. What is the diagnosis?

2. What further investigations are required? Give two.

3. What treatment is available?

Answers overleaf

1. 1. Hyperthyroidism due to inappropriate TSH secretion (as shown by high free thyroid hormone levels and inappropriately raised serum TSH). The vast majority of patients with hyperthyroidism have primary hyperfunction of the thyroid gland (Graves' disease or a functioning adenoma) which causes secondary suppression of TSH secretion. 'Secondary' TSH-driven hyperthyroidism is rare. Causes include pituitary tumours secreting TSH, the 'inappropriate' TSH hypersecretion syndrome, and production of TSH or related peptides by trophoblastic tumours. TSH-secreting pituitary tumours (usually a macroadenoma) may also secrete multiple hormones (GH, ACTH, LH/FSH, and prolactin) as well as excess amounts of the glycoprotein alpha subunit common to TSH, LH and FSH (and also HCG). Therefore, the alpha subunit/TSH ratio is >1.0. As TSH secretion by these tumours is autonomous, TSH levels are unaffected by normal stimulatory factors (TRH) or inhibitory factors (e.g. bromocriptine).

Inappropriate non-neoplastic secretion of TSH is due to reduced sensitivity of the pituitary thyrotrophs to the negative feedback inhibition of thyroid hormones. TSH secretion is further stimulated by TRH and generally inhibited by bromocriptine. The alpha-subunit/TSH ratio is <1.0, as in normal subjects.

2. Further investigations should include CT imaging of the pituitary gland to determine whether a tumour is present; measurement of TSH levels after TRH and bromocriptine; and determination of alpha-subunit levels and alpha-subunit/TSH ratio.

In this case, pituitary CT showed no evidence of a tumour; TSH levels rose after TRH and fell after bromocriptine, and the alpha-subunit/TSH ratio was 0.8. Pregnancy test and pelvic ultrasound were normal, excluding trophoblastic disease. The diagnosis was therefore inappropriate TSH hypersecretion.

3. TSH-secreting pituitary tumours may require surgical removal if large or threatening vision. Somatostatin analogues may reduce TSH secretion both from adenomas and in the non-neoplastic syndrome, and bromocriptine or a modified T3 derivative may be useful in the latter. Antithyroid drugs and thyroidectomy are generally ineffective because continuing TSH hypersecretion stimulates both thyroid hormone output and re-growth of the gland.

2. A 36 year old woman presented with muscle weakness, cramps numbness and tingling of the hands and feet. Hypertension had been diagnosed four years previously after the birth of her last child. She was taking one tablet of Tenoretic (atenolol and chlorthalidone) every morning. She denied vomiting, diarrhoea, or laxative abuse. There was no family history of hypertension.

On examination, her pulse was regular at 60 beats/min, BP 150/100 mm Hg supine, BP 155/100 mm Hg standing. While the blood pressure was being measured, she developed Trousseau's sign. The chest, heart and abdomen were normal. There was mild weakness of the proximal muscles, but no abnormalities in sensation or the reflexes. Fundoscopy was normal.

Investigations showed:

FBC normal

After withdrawal of treatment:

Plasma	sodium	145 mmol/l
	potassium	2.8 mmol/l
	chloride	100 mmol/l
	urea	4.5 mmol/l
Serum	creatinine	83 μmol/l
	calcium	2.4 mmol/l
	magnesium	0.8 mmol/l
Arterial blood gases	pH	7.46
	pCO_2	3.2 kPa
	pO_2	13.6 kPa
	HCO_3	32 mmol/l
Chest X-ray	no cardiomegaly	
Electrocardiogram	prolonged Q-T interval and U waves	

Questions:

1. What are the possible causes of this patient's hypokalaemia?

2. Suggest two further non-invasive confirmatory investigations.

3. Name one invasive confirmatory investigation.

Answers overleaf

2. 1. Hypertension in a young person (<40 years of age) is more likely to have an underlying treatable cause than if it occurs in an older person. However, most cases still have essential hypertension. The presence of hypokalaemia (which caused this patient's muscle weakness and tetany) in any hypertensive patient should immediately raise the possibility of hyperaldosteronism. However, hypokalaemia is more commonly due to diuretic therapy, which should therefore be discontinued for 3 weeks and the electrolytes re-checked. The presence of hypokalaemia while following a high-sodium diet (for example 1.2 gram/day Slow Sodium) is presumptive evidence of primary hyperaldosteronism.

2. Measurements of plasma aldosterone and renin. In primary hyperaldosteronism, the increased production of aldosterone may be derived from either an adrenal adenoma or bilateral hyperplasia of the adrenal zona glomerulosa. Plasma renin will be suppressed in both conditions. Measurement of plasma aldosterone may distinguish between adenoma and hyperplasia, which differ in the degree of aldosterone elevation and the response to postural change. In normal subjects, standing upright activates the renin-angiotensin-aldosterone (RAA) axis. Patients with adrenal adenoma have increased plasma aldosterone levels when recumbent, which may show a paradoxical fall on standing. Patients with adrenal hyperplasia almost always show a rise in aldosterone levels on standing. All renin and aldosterone measurements should be done under conditions of salt loading, which will tend to suppress the RAA axis.

    CT scanning of the abdomen can detect adenomas measuring more than 1 cm in diameter. Magnetic resonance scans may offer greater resolution and precision. This patient's CT scan showed an enlarged right adrenal gland.

3. Selective adrenal vein catheterisation will show increased aldosterone concentrations on the side of the adrenal adenoma with low or normal values on the other side (where the gland's activity will be suppressed by sodium and water retention). These differences may be highlighted by comparing the ratios of aldosterone to cortisol on each side; cortisol secretion from both glands will be comparable. Elevated aldosterone values (or aldosterone/cortisol ratios) on both sides suggest adrenal hyperplasia.

3. A 64 year old woman presented with a one-month history of anorexia, pain in the epigastrium and left renal angle, 3 kg weight loss, increased thirst, polyuria and nocturia. Hypertension had been diagnosed 10 years previously and she was taking Secadrex (acebutolol and hydrochlorothiazide) as her only medication. She had been a life-long non-smoker.

On examination, pulse 60/min regular, BP 150/80 mm Hg. The lungs and heart were normal. She was tender in the epigastric area, but the liver and spleen were not palpable. The breasts were normal and there was no lymphadenopathy.

Investigations showed:

Hb	12.2 g/dl
WBC	3.5×10^9/l, normal differential
Platelets	119×10^9/l
ESR	19 mm in the first hour
Urine calcium	8 mmol/24 hours (NR 2–6)
Serum calcium	3.95 mmol/l
phosphate	0.83 mmol/l
alkaline phosphatase	88 iu/l
albumin	40 g/l
globulins	27 g/l

Parathyroid hormone (PTH): 33 pmol/l (normal range 29–85)

Questions:

1. What are the possible causes of this patient's hypercalcaemia?

2. Give two useful investigations.

3. How would you treat the hypercalcaemia?

3. 1. Primary hyperparathyroidism is unlikely in view of the border-line low serum phosphate and low to normal PTH levels. The normal ESR and globulins are against the diagnosis of multiple myeloma. A normal chest X-ray would be unusual in sarcoidosis. Thiazides may aggravate hypercalcaemia by increasing calcium reabsorption but would not cause hypercalcaemia of this degree.

Hypercalcaemia of this magnitude is highly suggestive of malignancy. In two large hospital surveys on hypercalcaemia, malignant disease (especially of the lung and breast) was the most common cause and accounted for over 50% of all cases in both studies.

2. Abdominal ultrasound·or CT scanning.

Abdominal ultrasound was performed because of the persistent pain in her left flank (hypercalcaemia on its own can cause both peptic ulceration and non-specific abdominal pain). This showed a large mass in the upper pole of the left kidney and multiple poor-echogenic areas in the liver suggestive of metastases. Histology of the renal mass subsequently showed non-Hodgkin's lymphoma; bone marrow examination was normal. Hypercalcaemia complicates 1–2% of cases of lymphoma; some of these tumours may be producing 1,25 hydroxyvitamin D.

3. Hypercalcaemia interferes with renal distal tubular function and impairs the responsiveness of the collecting ducts to antidiuretic hormone. The resulting diuresis and volume depletion increases proximal tubular reabsorption of sodium and calcium, and worsens the existing hypercalcaemia. Simple rehydration with intravenous saline (2–3 litres in 6–8 hours, if cardiac and renal function permit), will increase glomerular filtration and usually lowers blood calcium levels significantly. Addition of frusemide (which increases renal calcium clearance), but not thiazides, is also useful. Other treatment options include intravenous aminohydroxypropylidene diphosphonate, calcitonin, and mithramycin. Corticosteroids are useful in the hypercalcaemia of myeloma but are less effective in other malignancies.

4. A 48 year old farmer presented with a 10-month history of muscle weakness, easy bruising, backache, headaches and depression. He was teetotal, a lifelong non-smoker, and had previously been healthy. His only medication was a non-steroidal anti-inflammatory agent for vague pain in the ribs.

On examination, he had a plethoric face and marked truncal obesity with an obvious 'buffalo' hump. The skin was thin and bruised easily. The abdomen was prominent and showed pink cutaneous striae. The patient's BP was 180/100 mm Hg, pulse 80/min. The arms and legs were generally thin due to muscle wasting. He had marked weakness of the pelvic girdle muscles and was unable to stand up from a squatting position. The visual fields on confrontation were normal and fundoscopy showed arterio-venous nipping only. There were no abnormalities of sensation and the reflexes were normal.

Investigations showed:

Hb		14.6 g/dl
WBC		6.3×10^9/l
Plasma	sodium	142 mmol/l
	potassium	3.1 mmol/l
	urea	6.3 mmol/l
Serum	creatinine	86 μmol/l
	creatine kinase	68 iu/l
Blood glucose (fasting)		5.0 mmol/l
Chest X-ray		multiple rib fractures with prominent callus formation

Thyroid function tests	normal

9 am cortisol	933 nmol/l (normal range 220–720)
9 am ACTH	76 ng/l (normal range 20–80)
Midnight cortisol	874 nmol/l
Midnight ACTH	67 ng/l

Urinary free cortisol (μmol/24 hours): 1267, 1334, 1231
 (normal range <350)
Low dose dexamethasone test (0.5 mg 6-hourly):

9 am cortisol	874 nmol/l
urinary cortisol	1432 μmol/24 h

Continued overleaf

High dose dexamethasone test (2 mg 6-hourly):
    9 am cortisol   641 nmol/l
    urinary cortisol   823 µmol/24 h

CT pituitary scan: normal
CT adrenal scan: bilateral adrenal enlargement

Questions:

1. What is the diagnosis?

2. Name two confirmatory investigations.

3. What is the treatment?

Answers overleaf

4. 1. Cushing's syndrome. He has most of the clinical features of cortisol excess, including truncal obesity, atrophic skin, easy bruising, myopathy, hypertension, and rib fractures with prominent callus formation.

Serum cortisol levels are elevated, with loss of diurnal rhythm. The 'normal' ACTH makes ectopic ACTH secretion unlikely, as much higher values would be expected. Conversely, ACTH secretion is suppressed when an adrenal adenoma is the source of the cortisol excess. In cases driven by a pituitary adenoma producing ACTH (i.e. Cushing's disease), ACTH levels are within or somewhat above the normal range.

Suppression of 9 am cortisol levels to less than 50% of the basal value by high dose dexamethasone is compatible with pituitary-dependent Cushing's syndrome. Failure of suppression suggests an adrenal cause or ectopic ACTH syndrome. In this patient, high dose dexamethasone test produced an equivocal result (30% suppression in 9 am cortisol).

2. CT scanning was normal (as is the case in 75% of Cushing's disease), but higher resolution magnetic resonance scans of the pituitary showed a microadenoma. The source of ACTH secretion can be accurately located by selective venous sampling from the inferior petrosal sinus which drains the pituitary.

3. Exploration of the pituitary by the transphenoidal route and selective removal of the adenoma. Bilateral adrenalectomy is undesirable in pituitary-dependent Cushing's disease because of the risks of developing Nelson's syndrome. Metyrapone (which blocks cortisol synthesis) may be given to patients unfit for surgery.

5. A 64 year old woman presented to the casualty department following a grand mal fit at home. In the casualty department she had another two grand mal fits without regaining consciousness between them. Moduretic (amiloride and hydrochlorothiazide) had been started a month previously for hypertension but she was otherwise healthy.

On examination, she was drowsy and disorientated. There were no signs of meningism or neurological deficit, and her fundi were normal. The chest, heart, and abdomen were normal. Pulse 80/min, BP 160/100 mm Hg, temperature 37°C.

Investigations showed:

Hb		14.3 g/dl
WBC		$10.2 \times 10^9/l$
Platelets		$320 \times 10^9/l$
Serum	creatinine	90 μmol/l
	osmolality	246 mOsmol/kg
Plasma	sodium	104 mmol/l
	potassium	3.2 mmol/l
	urea	4.4 mmol/l
Blood	sugar	7.7 mmol/l
	lipids	normal
Urine osmolality		644 mOsmol/kg
Chest X-ray		normal
CT brain scan		normal

Questions:

1. What is the most likely diagnosis?

2. What is the treatment?

Answers overleaf

5. 1. Syndrome of inappropriate ADH secretion (SIADH). SIADH refers to a large number of conditions in which vasopressin (ADH) levels are inappropriately high in the presence of plasma hypo-osmolality. Causes of SIADH include drugs such as chlorpropamide, thiazides and carbamazepine which stimulate vasopressin release. It is important to exclude adrenal insufficiency before making the diagnosis of SIADH, as cortisol deficiency can prevent excretion of a water load. Very high levels of glucose or triglycerides can spuriously reduce measured plasma sodium levels ('pseudohyponatraemia').

2. a) Immediate measures: control of the epilepsy. This patient is in status epilepticus. Give intravenous diazepam (10–20 mg), but if fitting recurs give intravenous phenytoin (15 mg/kg loading dose, 50 mg/min) with ECG monitoring.

   b) Stop the diuretic. Restricting oral fluids to 750 ml/day will usually be adequate to allow the excess water to be excreted and the plasma osmolality and sodium levels to rise slowly over a few days. Hypertonic saline must be used with great caution because of the dangers of fluid overload and of central pontine myelinolysis which may develop if hyponatraemia is 'corrected' too rapidly. If simple fluid restriction fails, demeclocycline (1.2 g/day) or lithium (up to 1.8 mg/day), which produce a reversible form of diabetes insipidus, may be useful.

6. A 34 year old woman presented with an 8-year history of menorrhagia and anaemia. Symptoms of tiredness and inability to concentrate had caused her to lose her job. She also complained of cold intolerance, constipation and weight gain. She had no complaints of headache or visual symptoms.

On examination her skin was pale, cold, dry and scaly. The breasts were normal without galactorrhoea. The chest, heart and abdomen were unremarkable. Pulse 60/min, BP 120/60 mm Hg. Visual fields showed a bitemporal hemianopia. Sluggish relaxation of both ankle jerks was noted.

Investigations showed:

Electrocardiogram: bradycardia and low voltage QRS complexes
Chest X-ray: globular heart outline

Prolactin 3,600 U/l (normal range for females <700)

Gonadotrophins (follicular phase):
  Luteinising hormone   6.2 U/l (normal range 2.5–14)
  Follicle stimulating
  hormone   <0.5 U/l (normal range 0.3–3.0)

9 am plasma cortisol   519 nmol/l (normal range 220–720)
Total serum thyroxine   20 nmol/l (normal range (60–160)
Free T4   2.5 pmol/l (normal range 9.4–24.5)
Free T3   <1.0 pmol/l (normal range 2.9–8.9)
Serum TSH   >61.0 mU/l (normal range 0.5–5.5)

Thyroid microsomal and thyroglobulin autoantibodies: positive.

CT brain scan: an enhancing mass in the pituitary fossa with a suprasellar extension of 17 mm.

Questions:

1. What is the diagnosis?

2. What is the cause of the raised prolactin levels?

3. What is the treatment?

Answers overleaf

6. 1. Primary hypothyroidism and pituitary enlargement with optic chiasmal compression. The thyroid function tests show primary hypothyroidism (low thyroid hormone and greatly elevated serum TSH levels), and the thyroid autoantibodies suggest primary autoimmune thyroid disease. Severe primary hypothyroidism can cause pituitary enlargement through hyperplasia of the TSH-secreting cells (thyrotrophs) and in extreme cases can lead to optic chiasmal compression.

2. The hyperprolactinaemia in primary hypothyroidism is due to increased thyrotropin-releasing hormone (TRH) production by the hypothalamus, which stimulates both TSH and prolactin release from the pituitary.

3. The treatment is thyroxine replacement therapy, which will not only correct her symptomatic hypothyroidism but also cause resolution of her pituitary enlargement, visual field defect and hyperprolactinaemia.

7. A 28 year old nurse gave a 6-months history of episodic mental confusion, blurred vision, lightheadedness, palpitations and sweating. These symptoms occurred first thing in the morning, improved after breakfast, and tended to recur some three hours after eating. She has gained 10 kg in weight. Her mother has diabetes mellitus. Physical examination was normal.

Investigations showed:

Hb		13.8 g/dl
WBC		4.7 x 10^9/l
Plasma	sodium	142 mmol/l
	potassium	4.1 mmol/l
	urea	3.3 mmol/l

Liver function tests: normal.

Random blood glucose (measured by BM sticks on admission to the ward, while the patient was symptomatic): 4–7 mmol/l, laboratory blood glucose: 3.0 mmol/l.

After 12-hour fast (during symptoms): blood glucose 1.6 mmol/l, insulin 56.4 mU/l; insulin/glucose ratio >35 (normal range <10).

Questions:

1. What is the differential diagnosis?

2. Name one confirmatory investigation.

3. What is the treatment?

Answers overleaf

7. 1. She has hypoglycaemia due to excessive circulating insulin levels. The most likely cause is insulinoma; but administration of insulin or suphonylureas can also produce this picture. Factitious hypoglycaemia due to self-administration of insulin is said to be relatively common in medical and paramedical personnel.

2. C-peptide measurements. In hypoglycaemia induced by exogenous insulin, secretion of C-peptide is suppressed. Hypoglycaemia from other causes (e.g. large tumours metabolising glucose, or tumours producing insulin-like molecules which activate the insulin receptor) will suppress endogenous insulin secretion. By contrast, an insulinoma will continue to secrete C-peptide together with insulin despite hypoglycaemia. Measurements of proinsulin (the precursor molecule which is cleaved into insulin and C-peptide within the pancreatic beta-cell) provide similar information. In this case, high C-peptide levels during hypoglycaemia confirmed the diagnosis of insulinoma.

3. Surgical removal of the insulinoma. These tumours may be small and difficult to localise; methods include CT and magnetic resonance imaging; selective arteriography (which may show a tumour 'blush'); ultrasound scanning of the pancreatic head through the duodenal wall using a probe mounted on an endoscope; and inspection of the exposed pancreas (or scanning its surface with an ultrasound probe) at surgery.

ENDOCRINOLOGY : DATA INTERPRETATIONS

1. A 16 year old Caucasian girl presented with growth retardation and tetany. There was no history of steatorrhoea. She was on a nutritious diet and took no regular medications. Her sister had the same metabolic disorder.

   Investigations showed:

Serum	calcium	1.7 mmol/l
	phosphate	0.5 mmol/l
	alkaline phosphatase	661 iU/l
Parathyroid hormone		250 pmol/l (normal range 10–90)
1,25 hydroxyvitamin D		10 pg/ml (normal range 30–75)

   Wrist X-ray: cupping of metaphyses, widened and irregular metaphyseal lines.

   Question:

   1. What is the most likely diagnosis?

2. A 45 year old man presented with paraesthesia and numbness of his left hand.

   The results of his glucose tolerance test (75 grams orally, venous plasma sugar at 30 minute intervals) were as follows:

Time (min)	Venous plasma glucose (mmol/l)	Growth hormone (mU/l)
0	8.9	14
30	14.2	19
60	14.9	22
90	13.6	43
120	12.6	24

   Question:

   1. The two diagnoses in this patient are linked. What are they?

Answers overleaf
45

Data Interpretations : Answers

1. 1. The low serum calcium, low serum phosphate, and high alkaline phosphatase are all compatible with vitamin D deficiency. Causes of vitamin D deficiency include inadequate dietary intake (vegans) and malabsorption (chronic steatorrhoea). Anticonvulsant drugs may induce hepatic enzymes which metabolise vitamin D and inhibit intestinal calcium transport, and therefore lead to osteomalacia or rickets. The radiological appearances in this patient are characteristic of rickets. The most likely diagnosis in this patient is therefore type 1 vitamin D-dependent rickets, which is an autosomal recessive disorder characterised by a defect in renal synthesis of 1,25 hydroxy vitamin D. Tissue response to 1,25 hydroxyvitamin D is normal in the type 1 syndrome, but defective in type 2 vitamin D-dependent rickets. The hypocalcaemia is accompanied by secondary hyperparathyroidism which enhances renal phosphate elimination and causes hypophosphataemia.

2. 1. Acromegaly and diabetes mellitus. According to WHO criteria, a fasting venous plasma glucose of greater than 8 mmol/l or a value of >11.0 mmol/l two hours after a 75 gram oral glucose load are diagnostic for diabetes mellitus. In a normal subject glucose administration will suppress serum growth hormone (GH) concentration to less than 4 mU/l. In acromegaly, GH levels do not suppress normally and there may be a paradoxical rise in GH values following a glucose load. Approximately 20% of untreated acromegalics have symptomatic diabetes, and impaired glucose tolerance can be demonstrated in another 30%.

3. A 28 year old man has gynaecomastia. He is 1.90 metres tall (pubis to heel distance 97 cm, pubis to head 93 cm) and has an arm span of 1.95 metres.

Investigations showed:

Serum testosterone	4.6 nmol/l (normal range 10–30)
Plasma luteinising hormone	28 U/l (normal range <6)
Plasma follicle stimulating hormone	42 U/l (normal range <6)
Buccal smear: positive for Barr bodies	

Questions:

1. What is the diagnosis?

2. What is the treatment?

4. A 24 year old woman presented with symptoms suggestive of hyperthyroidism. She was on an oestrogen containing contraceptive pill.

Investigations showed:

Total serum thyroxine	186 nmol/l (normal range 60–160)
Free T4	12.5 pmol/l (normal range 9.4–24.5)
Free T3	11.8 pmol/l (normal range 2.9–8.9)
Serum TSH	<0.1 mU/l at 0 min and 30 min after intravenous TRH (200 μg)

Question:

1. What is the diagnosis?

Answers overleaf

3. 1. Klinefelter's syndrome. Patients with Klinefelter's syndrome show an increased lower/upper body segment ratio (normal <1.0), gynaecomastia, and subnormal development of the external genitalia (small testes and penis). The deficiency of androgens allows excessive growth of the long bones, and this is responsible for the increased arm span and long legs in relation to total height. Testicular biopsy shows fibrosis and hyalinization of the seminiferous tubules, which results in small firm testes and azoospermia. Chromosomal analysis shows a characteristic karyotype of 47 XXY, but some patients are mosaics with a chromosomal pattern of 46XY/47XXY and may be fertile.

2. Testosterone treatment, given by monthly depot injections, will improve symptoms of androgen deficiency, produce virilisation and prevent osteoporosis, but will not restore fertility.

4. 1. Triiodothyronine thyrotoxicosis (T3 toxicosis) is characterised by normal free thyroxine concentration and elevated serum T3. The suppressed serum TSH level and failure of a TSH response to TRH are compatible with hyperthyroidism. The oestrogen in the contraceptive pill increases the total serum thyroxine by stimulating hepatic synthesis of thyroxine binding globulin. T3 toxicosis tends to occur in patients with multinodular goitre and thyroid nodules, and occasionally in Graves' disease.

5. A 30 year old male patient presented with thirst, polydipsia and polyuria. The results of a water deprivation test were as follows:

	Plasma osmolality (mOsmol/kg)	Urine osmolality (mOsmol/kg)
9.00 h	289	115
12.00 h	304	120
15.00 h	308	116
16.30 h	308	124
DDAVP 2µg i.m.	306	124

Questions:

1. What is the diagnosis?

2. Name three causes?

6. The following results were obtained in an asymptomatic patient with hypercalcaemia:

Serum	calcium (corrected)	2.81 mmol/l	
	phosphate	0.8 mmol/l	
	alkaline phosphatase	100 iu/l	
	magnesium	1.2 mmol/l	(normal range 0.7–1.0)

Parathyroid hormone: <29 pmol/l (normal range 29–85)
Urine   calcium: 4 mmol/24 hrs (normal range <8)

Question:

1. What is the diagnosis?

Answers overleaf

5. 1. Nephrogenic diabetes insipidus.

   2. Causes include chronic hypokalaemia and hypercalcaemia; and drugs such as lithium, demeclocycline, amphotericin B, and methoxyflurane. There is also a rare X-linked recessive disorder which, unless treated early in life by high fluid intake and benzothiadiazide diuretics, causes mental and physical impairment.

6. 1. Familial hypocalciuric hypercalcaemia, an autosomal dominant condition characterised by enhanced renal reabsorption of calcium and magnesium, which produces elevated serum calcium levels in all patients and a concomitant mild hypermagnesaemia in 50% of cases. Familial hypocalciuric hypercalcaemia may be due to enhanced renal sensitivity to the hypocalciuric effect of parathyroid hormone.

7. A 40 year old woman presented with a painful goitre. The results of her investigations were as follows:

   Hb   14.3 g/dl
   WBC   11.2 x 10^9/l
   ESR   100 mm in the first hour
   Free thyroxine (T4)   32.4 pmol/l (normal range 9.4–24.5)
   Serum TSH   <0.1 mU/l (normal range 0.5–5.5)
   Radioiodine 131 thyroid scan: uptake at 4 hours <5% (normal
     range 6–18%)

Questions:

1. What is the most likely diagnosis?

2. What treatment is required?

8. The following serial cardiac enzymes were obtained in a 65 year old woman with worsening angina:

   Day 1 Creatine kinase 338 iu/l   Lactate dehydrogenase 327 iu/l
   Day 2 Creatine kinase 349 iu/l   Lactate dehydrogenase 319 iu/l
   Day 3 Creatine kinase 343 iu/l   Lactate dehydrogenase 334 iu/l

   Serum   TSH: 50 mU/l (normal range 0.5–5.5)

Questions:

1. What is the likely underlying diagnosis?

2. What is the treatment?

Answers overleaf

7. 1. Subacute thyroiditis (or de Quervain's thyroiditis), which may be viral in aetiology. Severe pain in the thyroid gland, made worse by swallowing, may be associated with fever and often a very high ESR. The hyperthyroidism is transient and is due to the release of thyroid hormones from damaged thyroid follicular cells. Endogenous TSH secretion is suppressed by the elevated thyroid hormones, and the damaged follicular cells are unable to trap iodine. Therefore, in the acute stage thyroid radioiodine uptake is poor and it may not be possible to obtain a thyroid scan.

2. The transient hyperthyroidism requires no treatment, but prednisolone may be useful in those patients with severe pain and systemic symptoms. Subacute thyroiditis may be followed by transient hypothyroidism, or rarely permanent hypothyroidism requiring treatment with thyroxine.

8. 1. Primary hypothyroidism. Untreated hypothyroidism may be associated with elevated creatine kinase, aspartate transaminase, lactate dehydrogenase, serum beta-carotene, and cholesterol levels.

2. Therapy should be started cautiously with small doses of thyroxine, for example 25 µg a day. Over enthusiastic treatment with larger doses of thyroxine may precipitate unstable angina or myocardial infarction.

9. A 50 year old male presented with weight loss, malaise, vomiting and diarrhoea.

The results of his short synacthen (ACTH) test (250 µg i.m.) were as follows:

Plasma cortisol at 0 min: 65 nmol/l
Plasma cortisol at 30 min: 224 nmol/l

The results of his depot ACTH test (1 mg i.m. daily for 3 days) were as follows:

Plasma cortisol Day 1:   156 nmol/l
Plasma cortisol Day 2:   367 nmol/l
Plasma cortisol Day 3:   783 nmol/l

Question:

1. What is the most likely explanation for these results?

10. The following results from a glucose tolerance test (GTT) (75 gram glucose orally, venous plasma sugars at 30 minute intervals) were obtained from a 45 year old woman complaining of increased thirst and general malaise:

0 min   4.3 mmol/l
30 min   11.8 mmol/l
60 min   5.6 mmol/l
90 min   3.7 mmol/l
120 min   4.5 mmol/l

Questions:

1. What is the abnormality in the GTT?

2. Name three causes.

9. 1. In normal subjects the basal plasma cortisol should exceed 190 nmol/l, and following a short synacthen test, plasma cortisol levels should rise by 200 nmol/l to reach a peak in excess of 550 nmol/l. The impaired cortisol response to a short synacthen test in this patient may arise from either primary adrenal insufficiency or secondary adrenocortical atrophy due to ACTH deficiency (from previous chronic corticosteroid treatment or hypopituitarism). In the depot ACTH test, plasma cortisol is measured 8 hours after i.m. injection of 1 mg synacthen depot on each of three consecutive days. Patients with primary adrenal insufficiency fail to achieve an adequate cortisol response to depot ACTH, whereas patients with secondary adrenocortical insufficiency show a stepwise increase in plasma cortisol to normal values (typically >700 nmol/l). The normal depot ACTH test in this individual suggests secondary adrenocortical insufficiency.

10. 1. Lag storage or alimentary glycosuria, which has a high early peak blood glucose with normal fasting and two-hour values.

2. Causes include gastric surgery, hyperthyroidism or liver disease. Occasionally it occurs in normal subjects.

11. A 42 year old woman presented with weight loss.

. The results of her investigations were as follows:

Hb		14.4 g/dl
WBC		8.9 x 10^9/l
ESR		18 mm in the first hour
Serum	calcium (corrected)	2.86 mmol/l
	phosphate	1.6 mmol/l
	alkaline phosphatase	156 iu/l
	TSH	<0.1 mU/l (normal range 0.5–5.5)
Fasting blood glucose		4.2 mmol/l

Question:

1. What is the most likely diagnosis?

12. A 56 year old woman gave a 6-month history of tiredness and weight loss.

The result of her investigations were as follows:

Plasma	sodium	132 mmol/l
	potassium	5.8 mmol/l
	urea	5.7 mmol/l
Serum	creatinine	78 μmol/l
	TSH	9.9 mU/l (normal range 0.5–5.5)

Short synacthen (250 μg i.m.) test:
   plasma cortisol at 0 min 78 nmol/l
   plasma cortisol at 30 min 89 nmol/l

Positive adrenal and thyroid autoantibodies.

Question:

1. What is the diagnosis?

Answers overleaf

11.   1. Hyperthyroidism. The hypercalcaemia in hyperthyroidism is due to increased osteoclastic resorption and increased osteoblastic bone formation. The elevated serum alkaline phosphatase reflects increased osteoblastic activity.

12.   1. The serum electrolytes suggest adrenocortical insufficiency, and the raised serum TSH is compatible with the diagnosis of primary hypothyroidism. The abnormal short synacthen test confirms the presence of primary adrenocortical insufficiency, which is usually due to autoimmune destruction of the adrenal cortex (Addison's disease) and the majority of these patients have positive adrenal autoantibodies. Addison's disease may be accompanied by thyroid disease (hypothyroidism or hyperthyroidism), diabetes mellitus, pernicious anaemia, gonadal failure, and hypoparathyroidism. This spectrum of endocrine disorders is termed the polyglandular failure syndrome or Schmidt's syndrome.

13. A 42 year old man presented with muscle weakness and haemoptysis.

Investigations showed:

Plasma	sodium	143 mmol/l
	potassium	2.8 mmol/l
	urea	3.7 mmol/l
Blood	glucose	13.6 mmol/l
Serum	bicarbonate	34 mmol/l

Question:

1. What is the most likely diagnosis?

2. Name two further important investigations.

14. A 29 year old woman presented with menstrual irregularity, excessive facial and body hair, weight gain, and infertility. Menarche occurred at the age of twelve. Vaginal examination was normal.

Investigations showed:

Serum	testosterone	2.6 nmol/l (normal range 0.8–1.6)
Plasma	17-hydroxyprogesterone	2.0 nmol/l (normal range <15).
	follicle stimulating hormone	5 U/l (normal range follicular phase <8)
	luteinising hormone	21 U/l (normal range follicular phase <6)
Urinary free cortisol		200 μmol/24 hours (normal range <350)

Question:

1. What is the most likely diagnosis?

Answers overleaf

13. 1. Ectopic ACTH syndrome from oat cell carcinoma of bronchus.
In these patients, plasma cortisol levels are very high and may
produce a profound proximal myopathy, diabetes mellitus,
increased skin pigmentation, and severe hypokalaemic alka-
losis.

  2. Chest X-ray. Serum ACTH and cortisol, before and after
dexamethasone and metyrapone.

14. 1. Polycystic ovary syndrome (PCOS). These patients present with
obesity, amenorrhoea/oligomenorrhoea, hirsutism, and infertility. Modestly elevated serum testosterone and a raised LH:FSH
ratio (especially a ratio >3.0) are suggestive of PCOS. Pelvic
ultrasound examination showed this patient had polycystic
ovaries, but cystic ovaries are also seen in other endocrine
disorders, such as congenital adrenal hyperplasia and Cushing's
syndrome (both may present with clinical features similar to
PCOS). However, the normal 17-hydroxyprogesterone excludes
the most common variety of congenital adrenal hyperplasia (21-
hydroxylase deficiency), and Cushing's syndrome is unlikely
with a normal urinary free cortisol.

1. A 75 year old diabetic man was admitted with a painful right leg. Examination revealed a large abdominal aortic aneurysm, an absent right femoral pulse and a swollen ischaemic right leg. He was being treated for hypertension with atenolol and nifedipine and his blood pressure was 180/90. He had evidence of diabetic nephropathy with a serum creatinine of 120 μmol/l and proteinuria of 4 g/l. An aortogram via the left femoral artery, demonstrated that the renal arteries were atheromatous but not involved in the aneurysm. The right common iliac artery was totally occluded and there was a poor blood supply to the leg via collaterals. A total of 100 ml of Conray 420 contrast medium was given. Following emergency aortic surgery, the leg was warm and well perfused, but the calf remained tense and tender. No fasciotomies were performed. Prophylactic flucloxacillin and amoxycillin were given. 12 hours post-operatively, he became febrile, hypotensive and sweaty and gentamicin was administered.

He was noted to be oliguric. The urine was positive for protein and blood with a sodium of 5 mmol/l and osmolality of 820 mOsm/kg. Microscopy revealed no organisms and no cells. Dopamine and mannitol were given and the urine output increased to 100 ml/hr.

Over the next three days his fever rapidly settled, he became normotensive and the swelling in the calf settled. However, he became progressively oliguric and the serum creatinine rose to 660 μmol/l. Physical examination was unremarkable except for the scars from his recent surgery and a purpuric rash affecting the previously ischaemic leg.

Questions:

1. List five possible causes of renal failure in this case.

2. Which of these causes do you favour and why?

Answers overleaf

11. This patient was given a high dose of intra-arterial contrast medium and was susceptible to contrast nephropathy as he was old, an arteriopath, a diabetic and had pre-existing renal disease.

He had several causes for acute tubular necrosis, including hypotension, probable septicaemia, aminoglycoside administration, and rhabdomyolysis.

Acute allergic interstitial nephritis may have been caused by the flucloxacillin. It is not always associated with a rash and should be suspected if there is eosinophilia.

Athero-embolic disease, in which cholesterol from a ruptured atheromatous plaque embolizes into the renal micro-circulation is often associated with evidence of emboli elsewhere, and may explain the purpura in the legs of this patient.

The ureters are occasionally damaged during aortic surgery. (They may also be involved in an inflammatory aortic aneurysm.) Although the left renal vein is often divided to gain good access to the upper part of an aneurysm, it is unclear how this affects the function of the left kidney.

2. This patient did not have established renal failure immediately post-operatively since his kidneys responded appropriately to hypoperfusion by retaining salt and water.

The most likely diagnosis was post-operative rhabdomyolysis because he had a positive stick test for blood, but no red cells in his urine, indicating myoglobinuria.

2. A 65 year old overweight woman developed low back pain which was particularly marked after carrying her shopping for long distances. Shortly afterwards, pain developed in both knees.

    She consulted her general practitioner who gave her some tablets and asked her to return one month later. At the second consultation, bilateral oedema of her legs extending to the sacrum, ascites and bilateral pleural effusions were noted.

    Routine urinalysis revealed:

Glucose	+
Protein	+ + + +
Ketones	Negative
Blood	Trace

Questions:

1. What is the most likely diagnosis?

2. Give three other explanations for a combination of heavy proteinuria and glycosuria.

3. How would you treat this patient?

Answers overleaf

2. 1. The distribution of joint pain in this woman is not typical of a connective tissue disease and in an obese woman the most likely cause of her initial symptoms is osteoarthritis. After her doctor had given her medication for this, she developed signs suggestive of the nephrotic syndrome and on dip-stick testing of her urine had nephrotic range proteinuria and glycosuria, indicating both glomerular and tubular disease.

The probable explanation for this is an allergic reaction to a non-steroidal anti-inflammatory drug (NSAID). Most NSAIDs have caused occasional cases of allergic interstitial nephritis, one of the features of which is renal glycosuria. In some of the affected patients, nephrotic syndrome secondary to minimal change nephropathy has also occurred.

2. Diabetic nephropathy frequently presents with nephrotic syndrome.

Proximal tubular re-absorption of filtered protein is sufficiently increased in severe cases of nephrotic syndrome to produce proximal tubular dysfunction, one of the earliest features of which is lowering of the renal threshold for glucose.

Drugs used in the treatment of glomerular disease may induce diabetes; these include diuretics, steroids and nifedipine.

3. Withdrawal of the NSAID will usually result in prompt resolution of the glomerular and tubulo-interstitial disease. Steroids may accelerate recovery.

3. A 50 year old woman with a right radio-cephalic fistula developed numbness and paraesthesiae over the right thenar eminence after 15 years of haemodialysis. She had also noted some weakness of her thumb, which was most marked during dialysis. Her only other new symptom was mild early morning stiffness and pain affecting her shoulders. There was an aneurysmal arterio-venous fistula over the radial aspect of the right arm with an easily palpable continuous thrill. The lateral part of the thenar eminence was wasted, and abduction of the thumb was markedly weak. There was loss of light-touch sensation over the tip of the thumb and lateral two fingers.

X-ray of her hands showed sub-periosteal erosions of the phalanges, peri-articular calcification of the metacarpophalangeal joint of the thumb and widespread calcification within the digital arteries.

The following results were obtained on a sample of blood taken immediately before dialysis:

Plasma	urea	19.0 mmol/l
	sodium	134 mmol/l
	potassium	5.0 mmol/l
Serum	albumin	40 g/l
	creatinine	1010 μmol/l
	calcium	2.5 mmol/l
	phosphate	1.6 mmol/l
	T4	64 nmol/l (70–140)
	T3	1.1 nmol/l (1.2–3.0)
	parathyroid hormone	2.8 μg/l (<0.8)

Questions:

1. Give two possible diagnoses.

2. How would you treat these conditions?

Answers overleaf

3. 1. The most likely diagnosis is carpal tunnel syndrome caused by β2-microglobulin deposition. β2-microglobulin accumulates in patients on haemodialysis and is deposited as an amyloid-like material especially in joints, subcutaneous tissues and the carpal tunnels. Clinical manifestations tend to become obvious about ten years after starting dialysis, and are particularly marked if dialysers made with non-biocompatible materials are used.

Alternatively, the patient may have a steal syndrome, with blood being diverted from the vasa nervorum of the median nerve to the fistula. This diagnosis should be suspected if the symptoms are worse during dialysis.

The radiological and biochemical findings are typical of a haemodialysed patient with under-treated hyperparathyroidism. (In end-stage renal failure, the serum T4 and T3 concentrations are generally slightly sub-normal.)

2. Immediate carpal tunnel release is needed. Local steroid injections are ineffective.

Steal syndromes are very difficult to treat. Banding of the fistula may reduce flow sufficiently to relieve the problem. If this fails, the fistula should be tied off if suitable vascular access can be created elsewhere.

4. During her first pregnancy, a 34 year old woman was found to have glycosuria at 12 weeks. She was monitored regularly and, although the glycosuria persisted, the blood sugar was always below 5 mmol/l. At 32 weeks, ankle oedema developed. However, there was no proteinuria and she remained normotensive. A normal infant was spontaneously delivered at term. The placenta was intact, but the membranes were described as ragged. She and the child were discharged home well on the third day following delivery, but three days later she was, re-admitted with brisk vaginal bleeding. Examination revealed a temperature of 38.5°C, a pulse of 120/min and a blood pressure of 170/110 mm Hg. The uterus was just palpable in the abdomen and appeared to have involuted normally. Plans were made for an examination under anaesthetic, but a grand mal convulsion occurred, following which she was unrousable.

Initial investigations showed:

Hb	4.0 g/dl
WBC	15.6×10^9/l
Platelets	12×10^9/l
Film	Occasional irregularly contracted cells
	Spherocytes
DAGT	Negative
Clotting screen	Normal
FDPs	Normal
Plasma urea	35 mmol/l
Serum creatinine	310 μmol/l

Questions:

1. What is the most likely diagnosis?

2. What is the treatment?

Answers overleaf

4. 1. The history and laboratory findings are consistent with a diagnosis of thrombotic thrombocytopenic purpura (TTP). There is no evidence of disseminated intravascular coagulation. TTP is initiated by inappropriate platelet activation and usually presents, as in this case, with fever, renal failure, neurological dysfunction, microangiopathic haemolytic anaemia and thrombocytopenia. Although there is rarely an obvious precipitant, there is an increased incidence in the six months following pregnancy.

2. Daily infusions of fresh frozen plasma (FFP) usually induce remission, presumably by replacing a deficient factor which inhibits platelet aggregation. In some patients, there appear to be circulating factors which activate platelets, and these patients benefit from plasmapheresis. Prostacyclin infusions, steroids, immunosuppressants and heparin are all of unproven value. Platelet infusions often exacerbate the condition and should be avoided, if possible.

5. A 21 year old medical student was on holiday in Venezuela when he became unwell with a fever and sore throat. He consulted a doctor who prescribed penicillin V. Two days later, he noted that his urine was dark brown, but he thought that this was because he had not been drinking much. After he had increased his fluid intake, he thought that his urine was slightly lighter in colour. Because his throat had not improved after a week's treatment, he went back to the doctor, who stopped the penicillin and gave erythromycin. Five days later, he returned to the United Kingdom and consulted his general practitioner on the following day. Physical examination at that time revealed resolving tonsillitis, bilateral cervical lymphadenopathy and tenderness in both loins. The blood pressure was 170/90 mm Hg.

An urgent urological opinion was sought. The urologist, on obtaining the above history, arranged for urgent phase contrast microscopy of a specimen of the patient's urine. This showed numerous red blood cells, many of which were dysmorphic.

Questions:

1. Give two diagnoses.

2. Give three investigations.

Answers overleaf

5. 1. Post-streptococcal glomerulonephritis (PSGN) is one possible diagnosis since nephritogenic streptococci are endemic in South America. However, several features argue against this diagnosis. Firstly, the onset of haematuria in PSGN is usually at least ten days after the beginning of the illness. Secondly, there was no response to penicillin or erythromycin. Thirdly, PSGN usually causes the acute nephritic syndrome and there is little or no evidence of oliguria or salt and water overload.

IgA nephropathy is a more likely diagnosis as it classically causes haematuria early in the course of an upper respiratory tract infection and it is the most common cause of hypertension in young adults.

2. A renal biopsy would be the most useful investigation to differentiate these two possibilities.

The serum complement is likely to be low in PSGN, and normal or high in IgA nephropathy. The serum IgA concentration is elevated in only some patients with IgA nephropathy.

A throat swab and the ASO titre might help confirm a streptococcal infection.

6. A previously fit 64 year old ex-smoker who worked in a brewery presented to a District General Hospital with a two week history of swelling of the ankles. Physical examination was unremarkable apart from marked peripheral oedema.

Investigations showed:

Hb	11.4 g/dl	Plasma	urea	21 mmol/l
WBC	Normal		sodium	140 mmol/l
Platelets	Normal		potassium	5.0 mmol/l
Serum creatinine	216 µmol/l		albumin	21 g/l
		Urine	protein	12 g/24 hr

Chest X-ray: Normal

Renal biopsy: membranoproliferative glomerulonephritis crescents in all glomeruli

Immunofluorescence: flecks of IgG, C3 and fibrin in some glomeruli.

ANA, antiGBM antibody, anti-neutrophil cytoplasmic antibody and C3 nephritic factor: all negative.

Diuretics and immunosuppression with steroids and cyclophosphamide were commenced. In spite of this, his serum creatinine rose to over 900 µmol/l and he was peritoneally dialysed. After two weeks, he became pancytopenic and the cyclophosphamide was stopped. He developed peritonitis, and so the peritoneal dialysis catheter was removed and antibiotics were administered. He was transferred to a renal unit where he was found to be febrile, salt and water overloaded and encephalopathic. A chest X-ray at that time showed cardiomegaly, upper lobe blood diversion and diffuse pulmonary shadowing. The steroids were stopped. Despite adequate haemodialysis and ultrafiltration, he remained encephalopathic and a new chest X-ray, two days after the first, showed increased pulmonary shadowing with an air bronchogram. He complained of a cough productive of white frothy sputum, and fine crepitations were noted at the apices of both lungs. Arterial blood gasses taken while breathing room air showed pO_2 45 mm Hg, pCO_2 32 mm Hg and pH 7.36. Sputum and blood cultures were negative.

Questions:

1. What non-invasive investigation would you do to exclude intrapulmonary haemorrhage?
2. Name two other possible causes of the pulmonary infiltrates.
3. What further investigations would you do to help establish the diagnosis?

Answers overleaf
69

6. 1. This patient has rapidly-progressive glomerulonephritis and there is an association between this condition and haemoptysis, first described by Goodpasture. Under a half of patients with Goodpasture's syndrome have antiGBM antibodies, and so intra- pulmonary haemorrhage is a possibility in this patient. This can easily be excluded by measuring the transfer factor which is raised in intra-pulmonary haemorrhage.

2. Intra-alveolar pulmonary oedema owing to salt and water overload is a potential cause of this appearance but should have improved with ultrafiltration.

   Pulmonary vasculitis should also be considered, but there is little evidence of a systemic vasculitis. The anti-neutrophil cytoplasmic antibody is neither very specific nor very sensitive for Wegener's granulomatosis.

   Infection is probably the cause of the lung pathology and, in view of the recent immunosuppression, an opportunist such as pneumocystis might be responsible.

3. Bronchial lavage or a lung biopsy will probably be required to establish the diagnosis.

7. A 70 kg man commenced regular haemodialysis in Newcastle in
    1980. Six months later he complained of pain in the shoulders and
    hips and difficulty descending stairs. He was taking aluminium
    hydroxide as a phosphate binder but was not on 1-alpha hydroxy-
    cholecalciferol. Physical examination confirmed the presence of
    proximal muscle weakness.

    Investigations showed:

Hb		6.5 g/dl
MCV		78 fl
MCH		24 pg
Serum	albumin	41 g/l
	calcium	2.55 mmol/l
	phosphate	1.1 mmol/l (N)
	alkaline phosphatase	normal (N)
	parathyroid hormone	low normal (N)

    X-ray hips : Looser's zones in both femoral necks

    Following a sub-total parathyroidectomy he remained hyper-
    calcaemic and his pain was unimproved. One week post-
    operatively, he was noted to have severe myoclonic spasms and
    marked asterixis.

    Questions:

    1. What is your diagnosis?

    2. How would you confirm your diagnosis?

    3. What is the treatment?

    4. What is the prognosis without treatment?

Answers overleaf

7. 1. This patient presents all of the features of the aluminium intoxication syndrome. Aluminium, added to reservoir water as a flocculating agent, is absorbed from dialysate and accumulates in dialysis patients because it is not excreted in urine as normally happens. Aluminium gels, prescribed as phosphate binders, contribute to the aluminium overload.

   Aluminium deposits in bone, reducing bone turnover and usually causing severe osteomalacia, pain and fractures. There is no response to either treatment with vitamin D or parathyroidectomy. A hypochromic microcytic anaemia develops, owing to interference with haem metabolism. Dialysis dementia classically presents with word-finding difficulties and myoclonic spasms.

2. The diagnosis can be confirmed by measuring the bone aluminium content. Serum aluminium levels are not useful unless the patient has been given desferrioxamine two days previously to mobilise tissue aluminium.

3. Desferrioxamine given at the end of each dialysis session will remove some aluminium and may lead to clinical improvement in mild cases. De-ionisation and reverse osmosis of dialysate to remove aluminium will prevent the syndrome developing. Aluminium-containing phosphate binders should not be used.

4. The prognosis is poor. There is rapid development of global dementia and death within two years can be expected.

1. A 30 year old hypertensive man treated with propranolol and Navidrex K was admitted for investigation of hypokalaemia.

   He had the following results (normal ranges shown in brackets):

Plasma renin activity (supine 1 hour):	0.8 ng/ml/hr (1–3)
Plasma renin activity (standing 1 hour):	0.9 ng/ml/hr (3–6)
24 hour urinary aldosterone:	51 nmoles (10–50)

   Questions:

   1. How do you interpret these results?

   2. How should the patient be investigated further to confirm a diagnosis of an adrenal adenoma?

2. Renal vein sampling performed on a 20 year old hypertensive woman with a loud abdominal bruit revealed a left-to-right ratio of plasma renin activity of 2.1:1. After two months treatment with maximal doses of enalapril the blood pressure was 190/120 mm Hg.

   Questions:

   1. What is the diagnosis?

   2. What is the likely response to surgical intervention and why?

Answers overleaf

1. 1. The patient has hyporeninaemic hyperaldosteronism, suggesting that he has Conn's syndrome. However, this diagnosis cannot be made confidently since he is taking beta-blockers, which inhibit renin release, and diuretics, which stimulate renin release. Hypokalaemia is present, which will tend to lower aldosterone production.

2. The drugs should be stopped for at least two weeks before the patient is investigated further. An aldosterone suppression test is probably the best way of diagnosing Conn's syndrome. Plasma renin activity (recumbent and ambulant) and plasma aldosterone are measured before and after salt loading with oral sodium supplements and fludrocortisone. In primary hyperaldosteronism, the plasma renin activity is low and fails to rise on standing, and the plasma aldosterone concentration remains elevated throughout the test. Selective adrenal vein sampling, measuring the ratio of aldosterone to cortisol, helps to establish whether there is a solitary adenoma or bilateral hyperplasia of the zona glomerulosa. Conn's adenomas are usually small and so ultrasound and CT-scanning may fail to identify their presence. Radio-labelled cholesterol scanning, performed during treatment with dexamethasone, is proving to be increasingly useful.

2. 1. The patient has a 'significant' left renal artery stenosis as the ratio is above 1.6:1. It should be noted that a high concentration of renin in one renal vein may reflect decreased blood flow through that kidney rather than an increase in the absolute amount of renin produced by that kidney.

2. There is likely to be a poor response to angioplasty. Unfortunately, neither the renal vein renin ratios nor the acute response to administration of an angiotensin converting enzyme inhibitor are of much help in determining the response to surgery. The best guide appears to be the response to chronic (at least six weeks) administration of an angiotensin converting enzyme inhibitor.

3. A 60 year old lady was noted to have radio-opaque kidney stones five years after having a terminal ileal resection for Crohn's disease. Because she had been feeling unwell she had been taking large doses of vitamin C.

    Investigations showed:

Plasma	urea	6.0 mmol/l
	sodium	138 mmol/l
	potassium	3.9 mmol/l
	bicarbonate	24 mmol/l
Serum	albumin	41 g/l
	calcium	2.6 mmol/l
	phosphate	1.0 mmol/l

    Questions:

    1. What diagnosis would you suspect?

    2. What other dietary history would you obtain?

    3. How would you treat this condition?

4. A 30 year old woman presenting with renal calculi had the following results:

Plasma	urea	6.0 mmol/l
	sodium	138 mmol/l
	potassium	2.9 mmol/l
	bicarbonate	13 mmol/l
Serum	albumin	41 g/l
	calcium	2.0 mmol/l
	phosphate	0.8 mmol/l

    Questions:

    1. What is the diagnosis?

    2. Give three possible causes of this condition.

    3. Will the parathyroid hormone concentration prove high or low?

Answers overleaf

3. 1. This patient has malabsorption syndrome complicated by oxalate stones. Calcium oxalate is normally formed in the gut, and absorption of oxalate in this form is poor. In malabsorption syndrome, however, much of the calcium in the gut is bound to fatty acids and so absorption of oxalate in the colon is increased. This leads to hyperoxaluria. Metabolism of vitamin C increases endogenous oxalate production and so exacerbates the problem.

2. Tea, strawberries and rhubarb are particularly rich dietary sources of oxalate.

3. Restriction of dietary oxalate and vitamin C intake, and oral calcium supplements are the main specific treatments of this condition.

4. 1. This lady has renal tubular acidosis. This is probably of the distal variety as neither nephrocalcinosis nor nephrolithiasis are common in the proximal form. The essential defect is of a failure of the distal tubular cells to maintain a large pH gradient between the blood and urine.

2. A congenital form of this condition exists but the genetics are unclear. A second group of patients have associated auto-immune disease and some of these have circulating antibodies specific to tubular antigens. The other large group of patients have various causes of hypercalcaemia, including thyrotoxicosis.

3. The patient will have secondary hyperparathyroidism. The exact mechanism of osteomalacia in this condition is unknown.

5. A 40 year old man who had had a terminal ileostomy for five years presented with renal colic. A plain abdominal X-ray showed no stones.

The following blood results were obtained:

Plasma	urea	7.1 mmol/l
	sodium	140 mmol/l
	potassium	3.5 mmol/l
	bicarbonate	16 mmol/l
Serum	albumin	38 g/l
	calcium	2.4 mmol/l
	phosphate	0.9 mmol/l

Questions

1. What is the most likely diagnosis?

2. What treatment would have stopped this condition developing?

6. Following lithotripsy, a 24 year old woman with recurrent renal calculi passed a number of small stones which on analysis were shown to consist predominantly of ammonium hydrogen urate.

Questions:

1. What is the likely cause of these stones?

2. What is the appropriate treatment to inhibit further stone formation?

Answers overleaf

5. 1. Uric acid stones are not uncommon in patients with ileostomies. The increased enteric losses of fluid and bicarbonate result in the production of a concentrated acidic urine, predisposing to the precipitation of uric acid.

   2. Regular ingestion of sodium bicarbonate supplements usually prevents the problem.

6. 1. Chronic infection with a urease-producing organism, such as *Proteus sp.*, Ammonia produced by hydrolysis of urea raises the urine pH and provides ideal conditions for the formation of urate stones.

   2. Continuous prophylactic antibiotics should be given to suppress infection. It is important to differentiate urate stones from uric acid stones, as the treatment for the latter (alkalinization of the urine) will exacerbate urate stone formation.

7. A 30 year old woman complaining of thirst had the following results:

Plasma osmolality	275 mOsm/kg
Urine osmolality after 18 hr fluid restriction	750 mOsm/kg
Urine osmolarity after 5 U of aqueous vasopressin	780 mOsm/kg

Questions:

1. What is the diagnosis?

2. What is the treatment?

8. A 20 year old Irish labourer was admitted to hospital unconscious. He was noted to be polyuric.

Investigations showed:

Plasma sodium	100 mmol/l
Urine osmolality	60 mOsm/kg

Questions:

1. What is the most likely diagnosis?

2. How would you correct the hyponatraemia?

Answers overleaf

7. 1. This patient has primary polydipsia. A 'normal' person generally achieves a urinary osmolality of over 1000 mOsm/kg after fluid deprivation and there is little additional response to exogenous ADH. In complete nephrogenic diabetes insipidus, the maximal urinary osmolality seldom exceeds 200 mOsm/kg. In central diabetes insipidus the urinary osmolality is usually low after fluid deprivation but rises by 200–300 mOsm/kg after antiduiretic hormone administration. Patients with primary polydipsia often complain bitterly of thirst during fluid deprivation, but are able to concentrate their urine moderately. There is characteristically no additional response to exogenous antidiuretic hormone.

 2. The correct treatment is to try to restrict water intake. Appropriate treatment should be given for any underlying psychological disorder.

8. 1. This patient probably has beer potomania. The minimum concentration of urine is about 60 mOsm/kg. Consequently, a high intake of fluids without a corresponding intake of solutes eventually leads to water intoxication. The most common circumstance in which this occurs is in habitual beer drinkers who fail to eat.

 2. Water deprivation corrects the hyponatraemia slowly and so complications such as central pontine myelinolysis are unlikely to develop. Hypertonic saline is dangerous in this condition. When the patient has recovered consciousness, he should be encouraged to improve his diet and stop drinking beer.

9. A 20 year old West Indian with known sickle cell disease developed nocturia and swollen ankles.

   Investigations showed:

Plasma	urea	8.0 mmol/l
	sodium	145 mmol/l
	postassium	4.0 mmol/l
	bicarbonate	22 mmol/l
Serum	albumin	21 g/l
24 hour urinary protein		10 g
Early morning urinary osmolality		310 mOsm/kg

   Questions:

   1. What are the two renal lesions?

   2. What is the link between them?

10. A 50 year old man who had had membranous nephropathy diagnosed 10 years previously presented with a rapid deterioration of renal function.

    Investigation revealed:

Serum	creatinine	1000 μmol/l
	albumin	20 g/l
24 hour urinary protein		15 g
Microscopic haematuria		

    Questions:

    1. What is the most likely diagnosis?

    2. How should this condition be treated?

    3. What is the prognosis if untreated?

Answers overleaf

9. 1. The patient has nephrogenic diabetes insipidus and the nephrotic syndrome. Damage to the medulla of the kidney commonly occurs in sickle cell anaemia and may lead to renal papillary necrosis. The cause is thought to be ischaemia owing to sickling within a relatively anoxic environment. Membranous nephropathy may also occur and usually results in the nephrotic syndrome.

Progression to end-stage renal failure has occurred. Interestingly, it has been possible to haemodialyse these patients successfully without significant haemolysis occurring in the extra-corporeal circuit.

2. Tubular damage releases tubular basement membrane antigens into the circulation, some of which are trapped in the glomeruli in a sub-epithelial position. Immune complexes are formed in-situ and lead to the glomerular lesion.

10. 1. Bilateral renal vein thrombosis has occurred. Thrombotic episodes are common in the nephrotic syndrome especially where membranous nephropathy is the underlying disease. The renal veins are affected to a disproportionate degree. The probable aetiology is urinary loss of anti-thrombin III. The classical presentation with loin pain, microscopic haematuria and an increase in proteinuria is due to venous infarction. In patients with an adequate collateral circulation there may be no symptoms. Renal failure may occur if both renal veins are affected.

2. The patient should be anti-coagulated. Heparin may be ineffective unless anti-thrombin III supplements are also given. Because warfarin is largely protein-bound, only a small loading dose is needed.

3. Pulmonary embolism is common and frequently fatal. Even with adequate anti-coagulation the chances of a return of useful renal function are small.

11. A 50 kg man with treated Hodgkin's disease presented with hypertension and the nephrotic syndrome.

Investigation revealed:

24 hr urinary protein	20 g
Creatinine clearance	150 ml/min
Urinary protein electrophoresis	Highly selective proteinuria
Serum anti-streptolysin O titre	700 U/l (normal up to 500 U/l)

Questions:

1. What is the most likely renal pathology?

2. What is the significance of the past medical history?

3. Why is the GFR increased?

4. What is the significance of the raised ASOT?

12. A 40 year old anephric man on haemodialysis had the following results:

Hb	4.5 g/dl
MCV	105 fl
MCH	38 pg

Questions:

1. What is the most likely diagnosis?

2. What investigations would help establish the diagnosis?

3. What treatment would you give?

Answers overleaf

11. 1. Highly selective proteinuria of this magnitude is suggestive of minimal change nephropathy. Hypertension is present in 10% of patients with this lesion and does not exclude the diagnosis.

2. There is an association between minimal change nephropathy and Hodgkin's disease, and so a search should be made for recurrent disease. There is an increased incidence of other tumours after chemotherapy, some of which may also be complicated by glomerular disease.

3. The major factors determining the glomerular filtration rate (GFR) are the hydrostatic pressure gradient and the colloid osmotic pressure gradient across the glomerulus. In the nephrotic syndrome, the colloid osmotic pressure gradient is decreased and this increases the GFR.

4. The anti-streptolysin O titre is a biological assay in which the in vitro ability of serum to inhibit haemolysis by streptolysin is assessed. Hypercholesterolaemia occurs in the nephrotic syndrome and some of the cholesterol is incorporated into the red-cell membrane. This expands the red-cell membrane, making the cell resistant to haemolysis. This is therefore a false positive result.

12. 1. This patient has iron overload complicating multiple transfusions. Renal failure causes anaemia for a number of reasons including relative erythropoietin deficiency, accumulation of inhibitors of erythropoiesis and reduced red- cell survival. Some erythropoietin is produced by even severely diseased kidneys, so that anaemia is much worse if the kidneys are removed. In such anephric patients, the major source of erythropoietin is the liver. This extra-renal production of erythropoietin remains under some degree of physiological control and so it is inhibited by blood transfusion, further exacerbating the anaemia. The resultant requirement for multiple blood transfusions causes iron overload which is reflected by a rise in the MCV.

2. The serum ferritin concentration has been shown to correlate well with total body iron stores in renal failure, and is regarded as the optimum parameter to measure. The serum iron and total iron- binding capacity are not good indicators of iron status in renal failure, and should not be used.

3. Desferrioxamine is given at the end of dialysis and some of the chelated iron is removed at the next dialysis.

13. A 30 year old man with a renal transplant developed a swollen great toe, for which his general practitioner gave him some tablets. Six weeks later he had the following results:

Hb	10.0 g/dl
MCV	110 fl
MCH	39 pg
WBC	$0.8 \times 10^9/l$
Platelets	$24 \times 10^9/l$

Questions:

1. What is your diagnosis?

2. What treatment would you give?

14. A 50 year old woman with chronic glomerulonephritis developed headache after 15 years of haemodialysis. Investigation revealed microscopic haematuria and a Hb of 18 g/dl.

Questions:

1. What is your diagnosis?

2. Why is it important to recognise this condition?

3. What further investigations might you perform?

Answers overleaf

13. 1. Allopurinol has been given to a patient already taking azathioprine. Azathioprine acts by inhibiting folate metabolism, and even in therapeutic doses causes mild megaloblastosis which is reflected by macrocytosis. Toxic doses cause pancytopenia. Injudicious use of the xanthine oxidase inhibitor, allopurinol, precipitates azathioprine toxicity by inhibiting its metabolism.

2. Allopurinol and azathioprine should be stopped. The bone marrow will gradually recover over weeks to months and during this period the patient may require transfusions of whole blood or platelets. Infections should be treated appropriately. Folinic acid may hasten bone marrow recovery.

14. 1. The patient has acquired cystic disease. Cystic degeneration of the kidneys occurs in most patients with end-stage renal failure after a variable time interval. It is most commonly seen in haemodialysed patients, but has also been described in conservatively managed, peritoneally dialysed, and transplanted patients. The aetiology is unclear, and the exact structure from which the cysts are derived is also controversial. The cysts may rupture into the collecting system causing haematuria or into the retroperitoneum, when pain is the usual presenting feature. Erythropoietin production is enhanced, explaining the rise in haemoglobin concentration.

2. There is a high incidence of neoplasia within the cysts and some of the tumours are malignant.

3. Specimens of urine should be sent for culture and cytology. Imaging of cystic kidneys requires great expertise if small tumours are to be identified. Ultrasound, CT-scanning and arteriography all have their advocates. Cystoscopy helps identify which kidney is bleeding. It should be remembered that patients with analgesic nephropathy have an increased incidence of urothelial tumours.

INDEX

Index

Index